All You Wanted Happ

VIKAS MALKANI

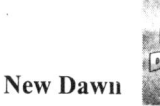

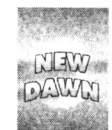

New Dawn

NEW DAWN
An imprint of Sterling Publishers (P) Ltd.
A-59 Okhla Industrial Area, Phase-II, New Delhi-110020.
Tel: 6912677, 6910050, 6916165, 6916209
Fax: 91-11-6331241 E-mail: ghai@nde.vsnl.net.in
www.sterlingpublishers.com

All You Wanted to Know About Happiness
©2001, Sterling Publishers Private Limited
ISBN 81 207 2388 0
Reprint 2002

All rights are reserved. No part of this publication may be reproduced, stored in a retrieval system or transmitted, in any form or by any means, mechanical, photocopying, recording or otherwise, without prior written permission of the publisher.

Published by Sterling Publishers Pvt. Ltd., New Delhi-110020.
Lasertypeset by Vikas Compographics, New Delhi-110020.
Printed at Prolific Incorporated, New Delhi-110020.

Contents

	Introduction	4
1.	Happiness	7
2.	Perfection and Happiness	11
3.	Make Peace with Imperfection	22
4.	Live Your Life Now	32
5.	The Power of Thoughts	85
6.	The Creative Nature of Thoughts	102
7.	Focus on the Positive	118

Introduction

The pursuit of happiness is the root motivation of all human life.

Beneath our so-called wants and desires for love, comfort, wealth, power, fame, etc., lies the unchanging quality of happiness — that all of us, without exception, seek — some consciously and most unconsciously.

However, it is imperative to recognize that there is no one absolute way to arrive at happiness — no one path, no one science, no eternal unchangeable laws. There are, however, hints and guidelines that can be followed, to hasten our journey and to make it smoother and less painful.

Happiness is essentially a product of a certain inner consciousness, which perceives everything in the externally manifested world. It is to make your journey to this happiness or inner consciousness easier that these practical hints and suggestions are presented.

They may be disarming in their simplicity, but if you accept them and absorb them into your inner consciousness, and put them into action, you shall be pleasantly surprised by their inherent power to transform your entire life.

The Author

Happiness

"Most people are about as happy as they make up their minds to be." So said Abraham Lincoln. It is not what happens to us in life that determines our happiness so much as the way we react to what happens.

On just having lost his job, Fred might decide that he now has the opportunity to have a new work experience, to explore new possibilities and to exercise his independence in the workplace. Whereas his brother Bill might, under the same circumstances, decide to jump off a twenty-storey building and end it all. Given the same situation, one man rejoices while the other commits suicide! One man sees disaster and the other sees opportunity.

I may have simplified things a little here but the fact remains that we decide on how *we* react in life and even if we lose control, that is a decision that *we* make.

Being happy is not always easy, though. It can be one of the greatest challenges that we face and can sometimes take all the determination, persistence and self-discipline that we can muster. Maturity means taking responsibility for our own happiness and choosing to concentrate on what we have got rather than on what we have not.

We are necessarily in control of our own happiness as only we decide the thoughts we think. None else puts thoughts in our mind. To be happy, we need to concentrate on happy thoughts. How often, though, do we do the opposite? How often do we ignore the compliments that are paid to us yet dwell on unkind words for weeks afterwards? If you allow a bad experience or a nasty remark to occupy your mind, it is you who will suffer the consequences.

I remember, when I was twenty-five, one day, I thought to myself, "If you are going to be a really happy person someday, why don't you start now?" That day I decided to be a whole lot happier than I had ever been before. I was stunned. It actually worked!

I then began to ask other happy people how they came to be so happy. Invariably, their answer reflected my own experience. They would say, "I had enough misery, heartache, loneliness and finally I decided to change things."

Perfection and Happiness

If we are unhappy, it is because life is not as we want it. Life is not matching our expectations of how it "ought" to be and so we are unhappy.

So we say, "I'll be happy when ..." Well, life is not perfect. Life is about being exhilarated, frustrated, sometimes achieving and sometimes missing out. As long as we say "I'll be happy when...", we are deluding ourselves.

Happiness is a decision. Many people live life as if someday they will arrive at "happiness" like one arrives at a bus stop. They figure that someday everything will fall into place, that they will take a deep breath and say, "Here I am at last ... happy!" Hence their life story is one of "I'll be happy when..."

Each one of us has a decision to make. Are we prepared to remind ourselves daily that we have only limited time to make the most of what we have got, or will we while away the present, hoping for a better future?

The following piece was written by an eighty-five-year old man who learned that he was dying. It is particularly relevant.

"If I had my life to live over again, I'd try to make more mistakes next time. I wouldn't be so perfect. I would relax more. I'd limber up. I'd be sillier than I've been on this trip. In fact, I know very few things that I would take so seriously. I'd be crazier. I'd be less hygienic.

"I'd take more chances, I'd take more trips, I'd climb more mountains, I'd swim more rivers, I'd visit places I've never been to. I'd eat more ice cream and fewer beans.

"I'd have more actual troubles and fewer imaginary ones!

"You see, I was one of those people who lived prophylactically and sensibly and sanely hour after hour and day after

day. Oh, I've had my moments, and if I had it to do over again, I'd have more of those moments - moment by moment by moment.

"I've been one of those people who never went anywhere without a thermometer, a hot water bottle, a gargle, a raincoat and a parachute. If I had it to do all over again, I'd travel lighter next time.

"If I had it to do all over again, I'd start barefoot earlier in the spring and stay way later in the fall. I'd ride more merry-go-rounds, I'd watch more sunrises, and I'd play with more children, if I have my life to live over again.

"But you see, I don't."

Isn't this message a beautiful reminder? The old man realised that in order to be happier, in order to get more out of life, he did not have to go and change the world. The world is already beautiful. He had to change himself.

The world is not "perfect". The degree of our unhappiness is the distance between the way things are and the way they "ought" to be. If we cease to demand things to be perfect, the business of being happy may become easier. We will then choose to have preferences for the way things might be, and decide that if our preferences are not met, we will be happy anyway.

As the Indian guru once told a pupil who was in desperate search of contentment, "I will give you the secret. If you want to be happy, BE HAPPY!"

You are Perfectly Imperfect Right this Minute

You always have been perfectly imperfect, you always will be. You will make mistakes on occasions, do things you wish you had not done, long for things you do not have. You are capable of honesty and sneakiness, kindness and hatred, compassion and cruelty. At the same time, though, you are a perfect living being, you have been entrusted with a life that is yours, to care for, enjoy and learn from. There is no one just like you. There never will be.

Many people have an unrealistic notion of what it means to be human. People talk about "having it all together," which is an illusory notion because we are always in a state of change. They think a day will come when they will no longer misplace their keys, lose their temper, offend other people, get scared, or feel at a loss for words. They might also think they will be able to stick to a diet, have a stimulating job that pays well, be liked by everyone, and wake up every day feeling bright and alert. If you really think these things are possible, look around you. Does anyone fit this description?

If you want to be happy, kiss these thoughts goodbye. When they come into your mind, smile at them without taking them seriously.

Remember, just because your head is full of the plentiful "shoulds", which gobble up your self-esteem, does not make them true. *Perfection is in truth, honesty, and kindness as we walk our path.* The goal is not to avoid slipping off the path, but to slide off with grace, enjoy the ride, and be kind to yourself.

Don't Sweat the Small Stuff

Often we allow ourselves to get all worked up about things that, upon closer examination, are not really that big a deal. We focus on little problems and concerns and blow them way out of proportion. A stranger, for example, might cut in front of us in traffic. Rather than let it go, and carry on with our day, we convince ourselves that we are justified in our anger. We play out an imaginary confrontation in our mind. Many of us might even tell someone else about the incident later, rather than simply let it go. Try to have compassion for the person and remember how painful it is to be in such an enormous hurry. In this way, we can maintain our own sense of well-being and avoid taking other people's problems personally.

There are many similar, "small stuff" examples that occur every day in our lives. Whether we had to wait in line, listen to unfair criticism, or do the lion's share of the work, it pays enormous dividends if we learn not to worry about little things. So many people spend so much of their life's energy "sweating the small stuff", that they completely lose touch with the magic and beauty of life. When you commit to working towards this goal, you will find that you will have far more energy to be kinder and gentler.

Make Peace with Imperfection

I have yet to meet an absolute perfectionist whose life is filled with inner peace. The need for perfection and the desire for inner tranquillity, conflict with each other. Whenever we are attached to having something a certain way, better than it already is, we are, almost by definition, engaged in a losing battle. Rather than being content and grateful for what we have, we are focussed on what is wrong with something and our need to fix it. When we are zeroed in on what is wrong, it implies that we are dissatisfied, discontented.

Whether it is related to ourselves — a disorganized closet, a scratch on the car, an imperfect accomplishment, a few pounds we would like to lose — or to someone else's "imperfections" — the way someone looks, behaves, or lives one's life — the very act of focussing on imperfection pulls us away from our goal of being kind and gentle. This strategy has nothing to do with ceasing to do your very best but with being overly attached and focussed on what is wrong with life. It is about realizing that while there is always a better way to do something, this does not mean that you cannot enjoy and appreciate the way things already are.

The solution here is to catch yourself when you fall into your habit of insisting that things should be other than what they are. Gently remind yourself that life is okay the way it is, right now. In the absence of your judgement, everything would be fine. As you begin to eliminate your need for perfection in all areas of your life, you will begin to discover the perfection in life itself.

Bless Today:
It Will Never Come Again

It is fine to work towards future goals, but do not forget that today will never come again. You have only twenty-four hours to enjoy it.

Some people put life on hold while striving for their dreams. At first their objective is, "After I attain_____, then I'll be happy." Then, later, after the success of attainment they are regretful. "Why didn't I take time to plant a garden?" (or to play with my children, to visit old friends, be kinder to my partner, relax, or go to the movies, or go hiking?)

Instead of waiting to be an old lady to wear purple, wear it now. Instead of waiting for retirement to live in a beautiful place, consider how to get there now.

So if you feel your life is filled with remorse and dissatisfaction, stop and ask yourself:

- What is missing in my life?
- What have I put on hold?
- What am I waiting for?
- What would really fill my heart and make me happy?
- What would I regret if I died tomorrow?

Though you may not die tomorrow, the saddest death is walking around like a robot, cut off from the magic of today — from love, from beauty, from being where you want to be.

A wonderful way to start the day is to bless it:

- Blessings on this day, may I make it special in some way.
- Blessings on my life, may I treat it with love and care.
- Blessings on all people, may I see the goodness in everyone.
- Blessings on nature, may I notice its beauty and wonder.

- Blessings on the truth, may it be my constant companion.

Learn to Live in the Present Moment
To a large degree, the measure of our peace of mind is determined by how much we are able to live in the present moment.

Without question, many of us spend much of our lives worrying about a variety of things — all at once. We allow past problems and future concerns to dominate our present moments, so much so that we end up anxious, frustrated, depressed and hopeless. On the flip side, we also postpone our gratifications, our stated priorities, and our happiness, often convincing ourselves that "someday" will be better than today. Unfortunately, the same mental dynamics that tell us to look towards the future will only repeat themselves so that "someday" never actually arrives.

John Lennon once said, "Life is what's happening while we're busy making other plans." When we are busy making "other plans," our children are busy growing up, the people we love are moving away and dying, our bodies are getting out of shape, and our dreams are slipping away. In short, we miss out on life.

Many people live as if life were a dress rehearsal for some later date. It is not. In fact, no one has a guarantee that he or she will be here tomorrow. When our attention is in the present moment, we push fear from our minds. Fear is the concern over events that might happen in the future—we will not have enough money, our children will get into trouble, we will get old and die, etc.

To combat fear, the best strategy is to learn to bring your attention back to the present. Mark Twain said, "I have been through some terrible things in my life, some of which actually happened. " I don't think I can say it any better. Practise keeping your attention on the here and now. Your efforts will pay great dividends.

Live Your Life Now

Do not put off living your life until you are "better." That is probably just the latest in a series of perfect reasons why you have not fully lived up until this moment. ("I'll do it when I'm older." "I'll do it when I've learned more." I'll do it when I find my soul mate." "I'll do it when I have the time." "I'll do it when...")

Regarding all those things you have put off until "later," keep this in mind: you are in your "laters" now.

Start doing the things you have always wanted to do and enjoy each moment by finding something enjoyable, *now*.

We are not talking about executing every grand scheme your imagination has ever created. ("I've always wanted to be ruler of the world.") We are talking about overcoming the tendency to say, "When my life is better, then I'll be able to start focussing on positive things."

We often form a habit of procrastination. Yes, we put off unpleasant activities, but we also tend to put off the enjoyable ones. We dole out pleasure, contentment and happiness as though they were somehow rationed. The supply of these things is limitless (as, by the way, is the supply of misery, pain and suffering). We do the rationing ourselves.

If you look, you'll find all the perfect reasons why you should not enjoy your life, why you should postpone enjoyment until certain things are different.

We say, the only thing that has to be different for you to enjoy your life is where you focus your attention. Look for all the positive things taking place in and around you right now.

As you find them, naturally you will feel more joyful.

In life we have either reasons or results. If we do not have what we want (results), we usually have a long list of reasonable reasons for why we do not have the results. We tend to rationalize (pronounced "rational lies"). All this is a waste of energy and a convincing argument that we cannot have what we want, which becomes another reason not to live.

We suggest that when you do not get what you want, rather than wasting time and energy explaining why you do not have it, find another way to get it. Focus your attention and look for all the positive things taking place in and around you right now. If you cannot find something positive about your environment, look again with "fresh eyes". Try another point of view. Be creative. What good are you taking for granted? If you cannot find anything, hold your breath. Within a few minutes, you will *really* appreciate breathing.

Whatever Anyone Says or Does Means Nothing About Your Worth

A great deal of my work centres on helping people realize that other people's opinions of them are simply opinions that come through their own filter. In other words, whatever anyone says or does means nothing, absolutely nothing, about your worth as a human being.

A person may give you useful feedback, have something valuable to say, but whether they like you, approve of you, or admire you need not affect your sense of worth or self-esteem. If everyone could internalize this belief, we could all relax and enjoy the show - the snow, the rain, the great big picture of life. We are free to feel joy when our self-worth rests quietly within us, not on the lips of others.

Unfortunately, many people live as if their self-esteem had a cord connecting them to external events and people. You receive praise, someone says you are nice or sends you a valentine and your self-esteem goes up. You do not pass your driving test, you get fired, someone is rude to you, your best friend forgets your birthday and your self-esteem goes down. This is the essence of a victim stance; you think the world is doing it to you. While you may have been victimized in your life, you are not a victim. You have a mind that can operate on your behalf by saying over and over: *whatever anyone says means nothing about my worth.*

An analogy that is sometimes useful is imagining that someone throws a dart at your arm. It cuts your skin, you bleed, and it stings. But you always have a choice about what you say to your heart and soul. You can hurt yourself further by saying : "He threw a dart at me. What did I do to deserve this ? What did I do wrong ? I must be a jerk and a bad person." Or you can also be kind to yourself by saying: "Ouch, that person threw a dart, that's not nice, that hurts. I'd better get out of here and get a Band-Aid and stay away from people who throw darts." So stop worrying about what everyone thinks about you because usually, they are not thinking about you at all, instead, they might be wondering what you are thinking of them.

Your Worth

Imagine that you were in charge of the care of a three-month-old baby. At feeding time, would you feed the baby with no strings attached? Of course you would ! You will not say, "Okay kid ! Unless you can do something smart or witty, unless you can sit up and say your ABC or make me laugh, you don't get a drink!" You feed the baby because it deserves to be fed. It deserves love, care and fair treatment. It deserves all that because, like you, it is a human being, a part of the universe.

You deserve exactly the same. You deserved it when you were born and you deserve it now. Too many people get the idea that unless they are as clever, smart, handsome, highly paid, sporty, witty as other people they know, they are undeserving of love and respect.

You Deserve Love and Respect Just Because You Are You.

Too rarely do most of us focus on our real inner beauty and our inner strengths. Do you recall watching "boy meets girl" movies? As the boy and girl struggled through thick and thin, you hoped and prayed the whole time that everything would work out. He went to war, she left home, he came back, she was gone, he found her, her brother told him to get lost, she told him to get lost, and all the time you hoped that they would live happily ever after. They were married and strolled off into the sunset as the curtain came down. You dried your tears and clutching your empty popcorn packet, strolled out of the theatre.

We cry at those movies because at our deepest level, we care. We love. We hurt. There is that inner core in all of us which is simply beautiful. Depending on how much we have been hurt, we will expose our deepest feelings, but we all share these qualities.

When we see the news stories which portray the plight of the people starving around the globe, we all ache inside for them. Each of us may have a different view as to how they can best be helped, but we all care. That is the way we are.

Accept that you have these qualities - the capacity to love and empathize and be human as you are human. Recognise your own worth and constantly remind yourself that you deserve to be treated well!

Poor Self-image Behaviour

Each of us must work continually on maintaining our positive and healthy self-image. The following behaviour traits are evidence that there is room for improvement in our self-image:

- Negative talk about ourselves
- Experiencing guilt
- Failure to give compliments
- Non-acceptance of compliments
- Not taking our own needs into account
- Not asking for what we want
- Starving ourselves of luxuries unnecessarily
- Failure to give affection
- Inability to receive and enjoy affection
- Criticism of others
- Comparison of ourselves with others
- Constant poor health

Change is difficult. The action of a poor self-image is always to perpetuate itself. As we start out on the road to self-improvement, the tendency is to keep replaying the old patterns of blame, guilt and self/denigration. Here are some suggestions for things that you can do to boost the way you feel about yourself:

- Accept Compliments - always say thank you or words to that effect.
- Give Compliments - one of the easiest ways to feel good about ourselves is to recognise the beauty in others.

- Always Speak Well of Yourself - if you have nothing good to say about yourself, keep quiet.
- Praise Yourself - when you do something right, give yourself a pat on the back. Acknowledge your value.
- Separate your Behaviour from Yourself - realise that your behaviour is not connected to your self-worth. If you do something silly, like smash into another person's car, it does not make you a bad person. You simply made a mistake. (Love the sinner, hate the sin).

- Treat Your Body Well - it is the only one you have got. Everything we do affects everything else. Exercise and nourish it well.
- Let people know how you expect to be treated - in particular, set an example by the way you treat yourself and them. Nobody should accept abuse from anybody!
- Get around good people.
- Work at having pleasure without guilt.
- Use affirmations.
- Read books which give you ideas and inspiration.

- Always picture in your mind how you want to be, not how you are. You will then necessarily gravitate towards your dominant thoughts.

Understand Separate Realities

While we are on the subject of being interested in the way other people do things, let us take a moment to discuss separate realities.

If you have travelled to foreign countries or seen depictions of them in movies, you are aware of vast differences among cultures. The principle of separate realities says that the differences among individuals is every bit as vast. Just as we would not expect people of different cultures to see or do things as we would (in fact, we would be disappointed if they did), this principle tells us that the individual differences in our ways of seeing the world prohibit this as well. It is not a matter of merely tolerating differences but of truly understanding and honouring the fact that it literally cannot be any other way.

I have seen that an understanding of this principle changes lives. It can virtually eliminate quarrels. When we expect to see things differently, when we take for granted that others will do things differently and react differently to the same stimuli, the compassion we have for ourselves and for others, rises dramatically. The moment we expect otherwise, the potential for conflict exists.

I encourage you to consider deeply and respect the fact that we are all very different. When you do, the love you feel for others as well as the appreciation you have for your own uniqueness, will increase.

Become More Patient

The quality of patience goes a long way towards your goal of creating a more peaceful and loving self. The more patient you are, the more accepting you will be of what you have, rather than insisting that life be exactly as you would like it to be. Without patience, life is extremely frustrating. You are easily annoyed, bothered and irritated. Patience adds a dimension of ease and acceptance to your life. It is essential for inner peace.

Becoming more patient involves opening your heart to the present moment, even if you do not like it. If you are stuck in a traffic jam, late for an appointment, opening to the moment would mean catching yourself building a mental snowball, before your thinking got out of hand, and gently reminding yourself to relax. It might also be a good time to breathe, as well as an opportunity to remind yourself that, in the bigger scheme of things, being late is "small stuff."

Patience also involves seeing the innocence in others. When I remember to see the innocence, I immediately bring forth a feeling of patience, and my attention is brought back to the moment.

I have found that, if you look deeply enough, you can almost always see the innocence in other people as well as in potentially frustrating situations. When you do, you will become a more patient and peaceful person and, in some strange way, you begin to enjoy many of the moments that used to frustrate you.

Be the First One to Act Loving or to Reach Out

So many of us hold on to little resentments that may have stemmed from an argument, a misunderstanding, the way we were raised, or some other painful event. Stubbornly, we wait for someone else to reach out to us—believing this is the only way we can forgive or rekindle a friendship or family relationship.

Whenever we hold on to our anger, we turn "small stuff" into really "big stuff" in our minds. We start to believe that our positions are more important than our happiness. They are not. If you want to be a more peaceful person you must understand that being right is almost never more important than allowing yourself to be happy.

The way to be happy is to let go, and reach out. Let other people be right. This does not mean that you are wrong. You will experience the peace of letting go, as well as the joy of letting others be right. Which will make them less defensive and more loving towards you. They might even reach back. But, if for some reason they do not, that is okay too. This will help you to be more at peace and have the inner satisfaction of knowing that you have done your part to create a more loving world.

Become a Better Listener

Effective listening is more than simply avoiding the bad habit of interrupting others while they are speaking or finishing their sentences. It also means to be content listening to the entire thought of someone rather than waiting impatiently for your chance to respond.

In some ways, the way we fail to listen is symbolic of the way we live. We often treat communication as if it were a race. It is almost as if our goal is to have no time gaps between the conclusion of the sentence of the person we are speaking with, and the beginning of our own.

Slowing down your responses and becoming a better listener aids you in becoming a more peaceful person. It takes pressure away from you. If you think about it, you will notice that it takes an enormous amount of energy and is very stressful to be sitting at the edge of your seat trying to guess what the person in front of you (or on the telephone) is going to say so that you can fire back your response.

But as you wait for the people you are communicating with to finish, to simply listen more intently to what is being said, you will immediately feel more relaxed, and so will the people you are talking to, They will also feel safe in slowing down their own responses because they will not feel themselves in competition with you. This will also enhance the quality of your relationships with them.

Everyone loves to talk to someone who truly listens to what they are saying.

You Don't *Have* to Do Anything

Whatever you do, do it because you choose to do it, not from any misguided sense of duty or obligation.

Sometimes people need to be pushed to the brink before they realize that this life belongs to *them*, not to the demands and desires of others. If you have a life-threatening illness, you are on that brink. If you learn that this is *your* life, you can more easily take a few steps towards de-brinking yourself.

Try saying this loud in your mind often: "I don't *have* to do anything." Say it a few times. Feel the sense of release, of freedom, or of unburdening!

You can add to it: "And what I choose to do, I can do."

Together they make a nice (and, perhaps, necessary) affirmation: "I don't have to do anything, and what I choose to do, I can do."

Avoid People and Situations that Upset You

Avoid things, people, situations and experiences you are averse to.

Some might call this cowardly. We call it smart. The world is brimming with things, people and experiences. We will never experience all of them.

So why not associate with the ones that naturally please you?

In some situations, it becomes difficult to reach a person (Mr. C) you would like to, without passing through others like Mr. A and Mr. B. In those cases, keep your eye on C. Keep reminding yourself why you are messing with A and and that soon you will be at C, and that C will be worth it.

Some examples of things to avoid: parties you do not want to go to, people you do not want to see, TV specials you do not want to watch (but think you should), movies everybody else has seen that hold no appeal for you, and so on.

This idea goes contrary to the claim that you grow through confrontation.

Yes, this is true. Tribulation and confrontation are great teachers. There is, however, quite enough tribulation presented to you *naturally*. You do not have to *seek* it, it will seek you. *That is* the time to practise acceptance, patience and forbearance.

If you can avoid the unpleasantness in the first place, by all means do so.

Of course, if you live in the freedom of your own thoughts and desires, you must also give the same freedom to others. Learn to accept the behavior of others even if it does not fit the pattern of your opinions.

Whenever you find yourself disapproving of another, examine your opinions. Explore your list of "shoulds" and "should nots." See your opinion as merely opinion, not truth, and therefore not worth getting upset about.

Others' opinions of you and your opinions of others are the cause of a great deal of unnecessary negative thinking. (All negative thinking is unnecessary, but the guilt, fear and resentment generated by opinions are particularly unnecessary).

Learn, in fact, to relish the differences between people. Imagine how dull the world would be if we all thought, spoke and acted the same way.

Become Aware of Your Moods (and do not allow yourself to be fooled by the low ones.)

Your own moods can be extremely deceptive. They can, and probably do, trick you into believing your life is far worse than it really is. When you are in a good mood, life looks great. In good moods, things do not feel so hard, problems seem less formidable and easier to solve, relationships seem to flow and communication is easy. If you are criticized, you take it in stride.

On the contrary, when you are in a bad mood, life looks unbearably serious and difficult. You have very little perspective. You take things personally and often misinterpret those around you, as you impute malignant motives to their actions.

Here is the catch: People do not realize that their moods are always on the run. They think instead that their lives have suddenly become worse in the past day, or even the last hour. So, someone who is in a good mood in the morning might love his wife, his job, and his car. He is probably optimistic about his future and feels grateful about his past. But by late afternoon, if his mood is bad, he claims he hates his job, thinks of his wife as a nuisance and believes he is going nowhere in his career. If you ask him about his childhood while he is in a low mood, he will probably blame his parents for his current plight.

Such quick and drastic contrasts may seem absurd, even funny — but we are all like that. In low moods we lose our perspectives and everything seems urgent. We completely forget that when we are in a good mood. We experience the *identical* circumstances - who we are married to, where we work, the car we drive, our potential, our childhood - entirely differently, depending on our mood.

When we are low, rather than blaming our mood as would be appropriate, we instead tend to feel that our whole life is wrong. It is almost as if we actually believe that our lives have fallen apart in the past hour or two.

The truth is, life is almost never as bad as it seems when you are in a low mood. Rather than staying stuck in a bad temper or an ill mood learn to question your judgment. Remind yourself, "Of course, I'm feeling defensive [or angry, frustrated, stressed, depressed]; I'm in a bad mood. I always feel negative when I'm low." When you're in an ill mood, learn to pass it off as an unavoidable human condition that *will* pass with time, if left alone.

A low mood is not the time to analyze your life. To do so is emotional suicide. If you have a legitimate problem, it will still be there when your state of mind improves. The trick is to be grateful for our good moods and be graceful in our low moods - not taking them too seriously. The next time you feel low, for whatever reason, remind yourself, "This too shall pass." It will.

Relax

What does it mean to relax? Despite hearing this term thousands of times during the course of our lives, very few people have deeply considered what it is really about.

When you ask people (which I have done many times) what it means to relax, most will answer in a way that suggests that relaxing is something you plan to do later — you do it on vacation, in a hammock, when you retire, or when you get everything done.

This implies, of course, that most other times (the other 95 per cent of your life) should be spent nervous, agitated, rushed and frenzied! Very few actually come out and say so, but this is the obvious implication. Could this explain why so many of us operate as if life were one great big emergency? Most of us postpone relaxation until our "in basket" is empty. Of course it never is.

It is useful to think of relaxation as a quality of heart that you can access on a regular basis rather than something reserved for some later time. You can relax *now*. It is helpful to remember that relaxed people can still be superachievers and, in fact, that relaxation and creativity go hand in hand. When I am feeling uptight, for example, I do not even try to write. But when I feel relaxed, my writing flows quickly and easily.

Being more relaxed involves training yourself to respond differently to the challenges of life. It comes, in part, from reminding yourself over and over again (with loving kindness and patience) that you have a choice in how you respond to life. You can learn to relate to your thinking as well as your circumstances in new ways. With practice, making these choices will translate into a more relaxed self.

Listen to Your Feelings (They are trying to tell you something)

You have at your disposal a foolproof guidance system to navigate you through life. This system, which consists solely of your own feelings, lets you know whether you are off track and heading towards unhappiness and conflict; or on track, heading towards peace of mind. Your feelings act as a barometer, letting you know what your internal weather is like.

When you are not caught up in your thinking, taking things too seriously, your feelings will be generally positive. They will be affirming that you are using your thinking to your advantage. No mental adjustment needs to be made.

When your experience of life is other than pleasant and you are feeling angry, resentful, depressed, stressed out, frustrated, and so forth, your feelings remind you that you are off track, and it is time to ease up on your thinking, as you have lost perspective.

Mental adjustment does need to be made. You can think of your negative feelings in the same way you think of the warning lights on the dashboard of your car. When flashing, they let you know that it is time to ease up.

Contrary to popular belief, negative feelings do not need to be studied and analyzed. When you analyze your negative feelings, you will usually end up with more of them to contend with.

The next time you are feeling bad, rather than getting stuck in "analysis paralysis," wondering why you feel the way you do, see instead, if, you can use your feelings to guide you back in the direction towards serenity.

Do not pretend that the negative feelings do not exist, but try to recognize the reason why you are taking life so seriously — why you are "sweating the small stuff." Instead of rolling up your sleeves and fighting life, back off, take a few deep breaths, and relax. Remember, life is not an emergency unless you make it so.

Love a Lot

Love is the most important thing in our lives. All the great masters, saints, and sages agree on this. But it seems to me that a lot has been lost in the translation of this teaching. It would appear that many of us have forgotten how to love, or never learned how to love, to begin with.

I believe I have learned one thing about love in recent years, which I will share with you.

I have learned that in order to love others, we have to love ourselves first. We do that by allowing ourselves to do things we love to do.

If you are feeling weak in the love department, the first place to start is with yourself. Spend some time figuring out the things you love to do, and the things that make you happy. Then start doing them. Do not expect things to happen overnight. It may take you a while, and you might need to get some guidance along the way. Fortunately, there is a wealth of information available today to help you do this.

Many times we have been taught that doing what we love to do is selfish or narcissistic. But, in fact, before we can give love to others, it is essential that we fill ourselves with love first.

Fill Your Life with Love

I do not know anyone who does not want a life filled with love. For this to happen, the effort must start within us. Rather than waiting for other people to provide the love we desire, we must be a vision and a source of love. We must tap into our own loving-kindness in order to set an example for others to follow suit.

It has been said that "the shortest distance between two points is an intention." This is certainly true with regard to a life filled with love. The starting point or foundation of a life filled with love is the desire and commitment to be a source of love. Our attitude, choices, acts of kindness, and willingness to be the first to reach out, will take us towards this goal.

The next time you find yourself frustrated at the lack of love in your own life or at the lack of love in the world, try an experiment. Forget about the world and other people for a few minutes. Instead, look into your own heart. Can you become a source of greater love ? Can you think loving thoughts for yourself and others? Can you extend these loving thoughts outward towards the rest of the world — even to people whom you feel do not deserve it ?

By opening your heart to the possibility of greater love, and by making yourself a source of love (rather than getting love) as a top priority, you will be taking an important step in getting the love you desire.

You will also discover something truly remarkable. The more love you give, the more you will receive. As you put more emphasis on being a loving person, which is something you can control, and less emphasis on receiving love, which is something you cannot control, you will find that you have plenty of love in your life.

Soon you will discover one of the greatest secrets in the world: Love is its own reward.

Realize the Power of Your Own Thoughts

If you were to become aware of only one mental dynamic, the most important one to know about would be the relationship between your thinking and the way you feel.

It is important to realize that you are constantly thinking. Think, for a moment, about your breathing. Until this moment, when you are reading this sentence, you had certainly lost sight of the fact that you were doing it. The truth is, unless you are out of breath, you simply forget that it is occurring.

Thinking works in the same way. Because you are always doing it, it is easy to forget that it is happening, and it becomes invisible to you. Unlike breathing, however, forgetting that you are thinking can cause some serious problems in your life, such as unhappiness, anger, inner conflicts, and stress. The reason this is true is that your thinking will always come back to you as a feeling; there is a point-to-point relationship.

Try getting angry without first having angry thoughts! Then try feeling stressed out without first having stressful thoughts, or sad without sad thoughts, or jealous without thoughts of jealousy. You cannot do it — it is impossible.

The truth is, in order to experience a feeling, you must first have a thought that produces that feeling.

Unhappiness does not and cannot exist on its own. Unhappiness is the feeling that accompanies negative thinking about your life. In the absence of that thinking, unhappiness, or stress, or jealousy, cannot exist. There is nothing to hold your negative feelings in place other than your own thinking. Remind yourself that it is your thinking that is negative, not your life. This simple awareness will be the first step in putting you back on the path towards happiness.

The Power of Thoughts

A simple thought. A few micro-milliwatts of energy flowing through our brain. A seemingly innocuous, almost ephemeral thing. And yet a thought, or more accurately, a carefully orchestrated series of thoughts — has a significant impact on our mind, our body and our emotions.

Thoughts have responses in the body. Think of a lemon. Imagine cutting it in half and removing the seeds with the point of a knife. Smell the lemon. Now, imagine squeezing the juice from the lemon into your mouth and digging your teeth into the centre of the lemon. Chew the pulp. Feel those little things (whatever those are called) breaking and popping inside your mouth. Most people's salivary glands respond to the very thought of a lemon.

For some people, the mere thought of the sound of fingernails on a chalkboard is physically uncomfortable. Try this — imagine an emery board or a fingernail file or a double-sided piece of sandpaper. Imagine putting it in your mouth. Bite down on it. Now move your teeth from side to side. Goosebumps?

Thoughts influence our emotions. Think of something you love. What do you feel? Now think of something you hate. What do you feel? Now, something you love again. We do not have to change our emotions consciously — just change our thoughts, and our emotions quickly follow.

Now imagine your favourite place in nature. Where is it? A beach? A meadow? A mountain top? Take your time. Imagine lying on your back, with your eyes closed. Feel the sun on your face. Smell the air. Hear the sounds of creation. Become a part of it. Feel more relaxed.

Most people who take the time to try these little experiments know what we are talking about.

Those who thought, "This stuff is silly. I'm not going to try anything as stupid as this!" are left with the emotional and physiological consequences of their thoughts — perhaps a sense of tightness, irritability, impatience or may be outright hostility. These people prove the point we are making, as do those who follow along with the "suggested" thoughts. The point being: thoughts have power over our mind, our body and our emotions.

Positive thoughts (joy, happiness, fulfilment, achievement, worthiness) have positive results (enthusiasm, calm, well-being, ease, energy, love). Negative thoughts (judgement, unworthiness, mistrust, resentment, fear) produce negative results (tension, anxiety, alienation, anger, fatigue).

Understanding as to why something as miniscule as a thought can have such a dramatic effect on our mind, body and emotions, helps us to interpret the automatic reaction human beings have, whenever they perceive danger: the fight or flight response.

Negative Thoughts and the Body

The fight or flight response puts a body through its paces. All the resources of the body are mobilized for immediate physical action—fight or flee.

All the other bodily functions are put on hold—digestion, assimilation, blood cell production, body maintenance, circulation (except to certain vital skeletal muscles), healing, and immunological responses.

In addition to this, the body is pumping chemicals — naturally produced drugs, into the system. The muscles need energy and they need it fast. Our body has armed itself to *fight or flee for its life*, and usually we just sit and seethe.

The repeated and unnecessary triggering of the fight or flight response puts enormous physiological stress on the body.

It makes us vulnerable to diseases like digestive troubles (ulcers and cancers at the far side of it) poor assimilation (preventing necessary proteins, vitamins and minerals from entering the system), slower recovery from illnesses (conquering a disease is far less important than conquering a wild beast), reduced production of blood cells and other necessary cells, sore muscles, and a general sense of fatigue.

The emergency chemicals, unused, eventually begin breaking down into other, more toxic substances. Our body must then mobilize yet again, to get rid of the poisons.

The muscles stay tense for a long time after the response is triggered, especially around the stomach, chest, lower back, neck and shoulders. (most people have chronic tension in at least one of these areas.) We feel jittery, nervous, uptight.

The mind always tries to find reasons for things. If the body is feeling uptight, it wonders, "What is there to feel uptight about?" Seldom do we conclude (correctly), "Oh, this is just the normal after-effects of the fight or flight response. Nothing to be concerned about." Usually we start scanning the environment (inner and outer) for something out of place. And, as mentioned before, there will always be something out of place.

The mind is a remarkable mechanism. Given a task, it will fulfil it with astounding speed and accuracy. When asked, "What's wrong?" it will compile and cross-reference a list of grievances with blinding swiftness and precision. Everything everyone (including ourselves) should have done but did not do is reviewed, highlighted, indexed and prioritized. All this is sparked by a sensation in the body.

Naturally, this mental review of negative events prompts a new round of fight or flight responses, which promotes more tension in the body, and more mental investigation into what is wrong?

Do you see how this downward mind/body spiral can continue

almost indefinitely? So when this downward mind/body spiral continues for a while, it is generally known as depression. But because depression, we hear, is a form of mental illness which is considered bad by our culture, we feel depressed about feeling that way, and a whole new cycle of the fight or flight response is triggered.

Considering all this, it is not surprising that some people make a decision deep inside themselves that life is just not worth living.

Negative Thoughts and the Emotions

The primary emotions generated by the fight or flight response are anger (the emotional energy to fight) and fear (the emotional energy to flee).

Contained within these two are most of the feelings we generally associate with the word *negative*.

Consider these lists:

ANGER	FEAR
hostility	terror
resentment	anxiety
guilt (anger at oneself)	timidity
rage	shyness (a general fear of others)
seething	withdrawal
depression	reticence
hurt (you are usually upset with someone else, or yourself, or both)	apprehension
	grieving (fear that you will never love or be loved again)

Any others you did care to add from your own repertoire could probably be considered a variation of anger or fear — or a combination of the two.

The problem with either emotion, in addition to the obvious unpleasantness, is that both tend to mar logical, rational, life-supporting decisions.

How often have you waded into a confrontation, only to find that, as the saying goes, you had stirred up a hornet's nest?

How many fields have you abandoned in your life? The field of a challenging new career? The field of a more fulfilling place to live? The field of relationships? (That's "relationships" as in "true love, a many-splendored thing.") The field of your dreams?

Because people are afraid of fear, they give up acre after acre of their own lives. Some find the snapping of twigs so uncomfortable that they abandon the territory of life altogether.

The Addictive Quality of Negative Thinking

For many, negative thinking becomes a bad habit which, over time, degenerates into an addiction. It is a disease, like alcoholism, compulsive over-eating or drug abuse.

A lot of people suffer from this disease because negative thinking is addictive to each of these three — the mind, the body, and the emotions.

The mind becomes addicted to being "right". In this far-less-than-perfect world, one of the easiest ways to be right is to predict failure, especially for ourselves. The mind likes being right. When asked, "Would you rather be right or be happy?", some people, who really take the time to consider the ramifications of being "wrong", have trouble deciding.

The body becomes addicted to the rush of chemicals poured into the blood stream by the fight or flight response. The thrill and stimulation of a serious session of negative thinking is something of a high. Some people "get off" on the rush of adrenaline.

The emotions become addicted to the sheer intensity of it all. They may not be pleasant feelings, but they are a long way from boredom. As the emotions become acclimated to a certain level of stimulation, they start demanding more and more intensity.

Negative thinking must be treated like any addiction, with commitment to life, patience, discipline, a will to get better, forgiveness, self-love and the knowledge that recovery is not just possible without following certain guidelines.

The Creative Nature of Thoughts

Thoughts are powerful. All the spectacular and terrible creations of humanity began as thoughts — an idea, if you will. From the idea came the plan and from the plan came the action and from the action came the object. Whatever you are sitting on or reclining upon began as a thought. The room you are in, and almost everything in it, began as a thought.

All the wars and fighting the world has known began with

thoughts. All the good, fine, noble and creative acts of humanity were conceived as a spark in a single human consciousness. The Eiffel Tower, the Mona Lisa, the Magna Carta, the Declaration of Independence, movies, books, television began in the human mind.

Even the creation of a human being began as a thought. As the old saying goes, "I knew you before you were a twinkle in your father's eye."

Victor Hugo described it this way — "An invasion of armies can be resisted, but not an idea whose time has come." Often misquoted as, "There is nothing so powerful as an idea whose time has come", it has been used so often that it has almost become a cliche.

Although we probably do not think about it often, it is easy to see that everything created by humans, both good and bad, began as a thought. (The categorization of "good" and "bad," of course, is just another thought.) The only difference between a thought and a physical reality is a certain amount of time and physical activity.

The amount of time and physical activity varies from project to project. Sometimes it is seconds, sometimes it is years, and sometimes the thought must be passed from generation to generation. Some of the great cathedrals took a century and three generations of stone cutters to complete. On the other hand, there was The Hundred Years' war. Leonardo da Vinci invented the helicopter four hundred years before one ever flew. Two hundred years ago, Thomas Jefferson envisioned a nation free from religious persecution.

Some people are particularly good at turning ideas into realities. Edison was one. Imagine: the phonograph, movies, an improved telephone and the electric light all from one man.

Henry Ford wanted to make a cheap, reliable automobile and invented the assembly line in order to do it.

Without thoughts, things that involve any sort of human action just do not happen. Where we are is the result of a lifetime of thinking, both positive and negative. If you wonder what your thinking has been like, take a look at where you are in life. Behold the answer!

If you are pleased with some parts of your life, then your thinking in those areas has no doubt been what you would call generally "positive." If you are not pleased with other parts of your life, then your thoughts about those areas probably have not been as positive as they could have been. The good news is that thoughts can be changed, and with that change come changes in manifestation.

Thoughts, if persisted in, can produce states of consciousness that, if persisted in, can produce physical manifestation.

If you persist in your thoughts of wealth, for example, this produces a consciousness of wealth — an overall state of being, that is open, accepting, abundant and flowing — and this consciousness of wealth tends to produce the physical manifestations of wealth: houses, cars, cash.

"But," someone once protested, "I don't have any money and I worry about it *all the time*." This person was proving the point, but in reverse. Worry is a form of fear, in this case a fear of poverty. This person, in holding an ongoing series of thoughts about poverty, created a consciousness of poverty, which created a lack of everything but bills, which caused more worry, and more poverty.

Positive thoughts yield positive results — loving, caring and sharing; health, wealth and happiness; prosperity, abundance and riches.

Negative thoughts bring negative results — dislike, indifference and withholding; disease, poverty and misery; fear, lack and alienation.

Our thoughts, in other words, create our physical reality. Where we put our vision - our inner and outer vision - is the direction we tend to go. That is our desire. The way we get there - well, there are many methods.

Why Do we Indulge in Negative Thinking?

Why do we use the power of our mind to create a negative reality? If our mind can generate health, wealth and happiness as easily as illness, poverty and despair, why are we not healthy, wealthy and happy all the time?

If a genie appeared and offered you a choice - health, wealth and happiness or illness, poverty and despair - which would you choose? If positivity is the obvious choice, why do we sometimes choose the negative? There must be something else, something deeper within us generating the impulse to think negatively.

Although you may have another word to describe the phenomenon, we call this wellspring of negative thinking, unworthiness. It is more than just a feeling or a passing thought. It is a ground of being, a deep-seated belief that "I'm just not good enough." Other phrases for it include insecurity, undeservingness or low self-esteem.

Unworthiness undermines all our positive ideas and validates all our negative thoughts.

When we think something good about ourselves, unworthiness pops up and says, "No, you're not." When we desire something positive for ourselves, unworthiness says, "You don't deserve it." When something good happens to us, unworthiness says, often with our own lips, "This is too good to be true!" When something bad happens to us, unworthiness is the first to point out, "See I was right all along. I told you so."

Some people cover their unworthiness with an air of self-confidence and an outward bravado bordering on arrogance. Their cover-up includes a self-indulgence and self-absorption that are almost selfish. These people, it appears on the surface, could use a healthy dose of unworthiness.

But, in reality, they are merely involved in a desperate attempt to hide — from themselves as much as from anyone else — the fact that they just do not feel worthy. They think the unworthiness is *true*, not just another illusion, and they respond by concealing it rather than laughing at it.

So where does unworthiness come from? A look at how children are raised might offer a clue.

Imagine a child, at two, three or four, playing alone in a room. An adult, usually a parent, is nearby. What for? To come in and praise the child every five minutes? No. For "supervision." The adult is there to be on hand "in case there's any trouble."

The child is playing and having a wonderful time. Two hours go by.

The child is "behaving" wonderfully. The interaction with the adult has been minimal.

Suddenly, the child knocks a lamp off the table. It crashes to the floor. What happens next? Lots of interaction with the adult, almost all of which is negative. Yelling, screaming ("This was my favourite lamp," "How many times have I told you?" "Bad, bad, bad"), and probably, for good measure, some form of physical punishment (spanking, deprivation of a toy, etc.). Almost the only interaction in two hours from the adult community was, "You are bad. Shame on you."

As an infant, we get unconditional, almost never-ending praise. Once we grow a little older and begin exploring our world, our primary form of interaction with adults—the symbols of power, love, authority and life itself—is usually corrective.

If we draw a picture, for the first time we get praise. But if the same picture is drawn again and again we are not praised but are asked to do something new.

Some children learn to do negative things just to get attention, because even negative attention is better than no attention at all. Being ignored, to a child, can seem like abandonment.

A part of us inside begins to add up all the times we are called "wonderful" and all the times we are called "bad". The bad seems to outnumber the wonderful by a significant margin.

We may begin to believe we are bad—that unless we do something new and remarkable, we are not going to be thought of as good; that we must strive, work hard and never disobey if we hope to get even a little appreciation in this world; that our goodness must be earned because we are, after all, essentially bad.

We may grow to believe this about ourselves, and from this fertile ground springs our negative thoughts. Sure, we have a lot of positive thoughts, but the negative ones tend to be more believed. A positive thought, checked against this belief of unworthiness, is labelled "false." A negative thought feels right at home. The unworthiness proclaims it true, and right.

Focus on the Positive

In any given moment, there is ample evidence to prove that life is a bed of thorns or a garden of roses. How we feel about life depends on where we place our attention — that is, what we focus upon.

Did you ever notice that every time you are given a rose, the stem is covered with thorns? (If you take the thorns off, the flower wilts more quickly. Florists know this and, therefore, leave the thorns on.) Do you say, "Why are you giving me this stick with thorns on it?" Of course not. You admire the beauty of the rose. Even if you prick yourself in your enthusiasm, it never seems to hurt — you are too involved in appreciating the rose and the person who gave it to you.

Right now, at this moment, without moving from where you are, you can find ample evidence to prove your life is a miserable, depressing, terrible burden, or you can find evidence to prove your life is an abundant, joyful, exciting adventure.

Let us start with the negative. Look at all the imperfections around you. No matter how good anything is, it could be better, could it not?

Look for dirt, disorder and dust. See all the things that need cleaning, repairing and replacing. An endless array of clutter, chaos and catastrophe assaulting your senses.

Now, let go of the complaining consciousness and look at the situation with an attitude of gratitude and appreciation.

Look around the same area you just surveyed and find the good. You can start with whatever you are sitting or lying on. It is probably softer than a concrete floor. Look at all the other objects you use but take for granted like glasses (both seeing and drinking), tables, windows, the walls and the ceiling sheltering you from the elements. Consider the wonder of the electric light. A hundred years ago, you would have to have been very rich or very lucky to have had even one. And today you probably have more than one - and a TV and a radio and many of the other electronic marvels of the age.

What around you do you find aesthetically pleasing? A painting you have not really looked at in years? The pattern on the clothes you are wearing? A flower? A vase? Wallpaper? Carpet? When was the last time you took a moment to appreciate colours?

Did you notice that you tended to feel better when you focussed on the positive things in your surroundings? The process of focussing on the positive to produce more positive feelings works the same with things more intimate than your surroundings — your body, for example.

If you look for all the things wrong with the body, pains here, bumps there, rough spots over here, too much fat; the list goes on then. But take a look at all that is right with your body. Even if you have a pain in your left foot, you can be thankful there is not one in your right.

To focus on the positive is not to disregard certain warning signals of a "negative" nature that, if ignored, eventually leads to inconvenience at best and disaster at worst. (If we use these "negative" signals to avoid disaster, then they are not so negative after all. Some even call them guardian angels.)

Let us say you are driving down the road and the little light goes on, telling you you are running out of fuel. We do not suggest ignoring that bit of "negativity" and focussing on how wonderful it is that none of the other warning lights are on. We suggest you get some fuel quickly.

Here, by the way, is where negative *thinking* can come in. The negative *reality* is that you are low on gas. Negative *thinking* begins the litany, "I wonder if I'm going to run out of gas before the next station. What will I do if that happens? During this inner tirade the driver, in his or her anxiety, usually speeds up, which only wastes gas.

What we suggest is this: take note of the negative information, decide what to do about it (whatever corrective action seems to be in order) and, while doing it, return to focussing upon the positive while working on "eliminating" the negative.

With medical conditions, it is good to keep track of symptoms, but it does no good to dwell upon them. The positive thinker might deny the early symptoms of a disease, making a cure all the more difficult. The negative thinkers might turn every mosquito bite into skin cancer.

Positive focusers take a middle road. They note symptoms accurately so that they can be reported to their health-care provider. They make an appointment. Beyond that, there is no point in dwelling on the symptoms, so they turn their attention to things more positive.

Have we made a clear distinction between *positive thinking* and *focussing on the positive*? It is a subtle but important difference. Positive thinking imagines any wonderful thing, no matter how unrelated it is to the actual events of one's life. Focussing on the positive starts with what is so, what is real, what is actually taking place, and moves forward from there in a joyful direction.

If you spend all your time in a positive future, when will you appreciate the present? The present is the future you dreamed of long ago. Enjoy it!

Slow Down

The speed of life on the fast track permeates every area of our lives. Hurrying becomes a habit. Even after we have simplified many of our daily routines, if we are still surrounded by fast moving people and phones that never stop ringing, slowing down can take a major effort.

Start by thinking about how you can slow down your morning routine. Getting up even half an hour earlier, so that you do not have to rush out of the door will make a big difference in the pace of your entire day.

Take the time to sit down for your morning meal. Eat in a leisurely manner so you can feast on each bite. Eliminate the distractions of the radio, TV and morning paper. Simply enjoy eating.

Make the gathering, preparation, and consumption of food a conscious part of your inner quest, especially if you have lunch or dinner in fast-paced restaurants away from the peace and quiet you have established in your home.

Plan to leave home early enough so you do not arrive at the office panting at the start of your workday. If you do drive, make a point of staying within the posted speed limit. Learn to appreciate moving with purpose at a leisurely pace.

Place post-it notes around your home or office to remind yourself to slow down. Over and over I found that rushing through a project meant getting it wrong and losing time in the end by having to do it over again, either partially or completely. Take your time and do it right in the first place, and enjoy the process as you go along.

Make a concerted effort to examine all the areas of your life, and figure out where you can slow down. If you have simplified a lot of your daily and weekly routines, you will not only have more time but can derive more pleasure from each thing you do throughout the day.

Slowing down will help you keep in touch with how you feel about what you are doing, and make it easier to connect with your inner self.

Figure Out What You Do Not Want in Your Life

In addition to figuring out what your priorities are, it is also helpful to figure out what you *do not* want in your life anymore. This is a subtle distinction, but it is an important one to make.

We allow a lot of mental, emotional, and psychological clutter to accumulate in our minds and our lives, blocking our access to inner peace.

This clutter includes doing things we do not want to do but continue to do, either because we used to do them or feel we should.

It includes spending time with people we no longer want to spend time with because we have outgrown the relationship or because they do not contribute to our inner growth.

It includes doing work we are not happy doing.

It includes trying to do too many things, even if a lot of them are things we do not want to do.

It includes not doing enough of the things we want to do.

It includes engaging in idle gossip and meaningless chatter that drains our energy.

An amazing amount of the clutter includes fuming over past events we cannot change, or being distracted by future events that may never happen. It includes judgement and harbouring thoughts that burn.

As you move towards developing harmony in your life, you will find that a lot of this stuff will fall by the wayside. Some things, however, will require an effort on your part to make sure they are eliminated.

Enjoy Each Moment

One of the ultimate objectives of attaining inner simplicity is learning to live happily in the present moment. Keep in mind that life is a continuous succession of present moments. Most of us spend an inordinate number of our moments regretting the past, or fidgeting in the present, or worrying about the future.

Worry and regret and being anxious, are habits that keep us locked in old patterns. But these habits can be eliminated once we have become aware of them.

If you find such habits are getting in the way of being happy, think about what you can do to change them. It sounds simplistic to say it, but you can get into the habit of enjoying your life.

Another way to choose to enjoy each moment is to start taking responsibility for your life. If you are not happy in your present circumstances, you have no one but yourself to blame. Make whatever changes you need to make so that you are happy.

Going within, will automatically bring you to a level of enjoyment of your day-to-day life that you may not have experienced before. Making the conscious effort to enjoy each moment will make your inner quest much easier.

Connect With the Sun

All the enlightened cultures of the past, and many sages of the present, recognize the role the sun plays in getting us in touch with our soul.

We know our bodies need the sun in order to maximize the vitamins and minerals we get from our food. Yet, we now spend close to 90 per cent of our time in artificial light.

Numerous studies have shown the debilitating effects on many people of the absence of adequate sunlight. Medical science has recently acknowledged the existence of SAD (seasonal affective disorder), and the need for sunlight for certain personality types.

One of the simplest ways to brighten your mood is to step into the sunlight.

Brief, definitely not extensive, exposure to the sun's rays is tremendously beneficial for our overall physical, mental and emotional health. But most importantly, linking with the sun increases our vitality and elevates our consciousness, thereby contributing to our inner growth.

Whenever you can, et ten to fifteen minutes of full exposure to the sun, either early in the morning or later in the afternoon. In winter, sit next to a sunny window to get a mini-sunbath.

Experiment with this. Connect with the sun every day for the next couple of weeks to see how beneficial it can be for expanding your inner awareness.

Rethink the Beliefs of Your Childhood

The number of people who have abandoned the religion of their childhood is legion. Many people are able to leave and never look back. Others leave, but are often consumed with guilt for doing so.

Some people spend years feeling angry and bitter about the restrictive, small-minded thinking they have spent their lives overcoming. And many continue to feel adversely affected, sometimes unconsciously, by the dogma and the belief systems that permeated their minds as children.

There are also those who never had a childhood religion to leave behind, and who still basically believe in nothing. And there are those who have allowed the predominant conclusion of pseudo-science — which says if we cannot prove it, it does not exist — to rule their thinking.

If you are beginning to take a look at your life, this might be a good time to examine any feelings you may have about the teachings of your childhood that could be holding you back from questions you really want to explore.

As you start to slow down and enjoy the silence and the solitude, as you learn to listen and begin to trust your intitution, as you start to make the changes in your lifestyle and habit patterns that will enable you to connect with your own truth, you will begin to experience a new way of looking at life and the world and your place in it.

Rethink Your Current Beliefs

While you are rethinking the beliefs of your childhood, do not forget to examine your current beliefs, the ones you may have acquired after you let go of the beliefs of your childhood, the ones you moved into at the time of your mid-life crisis, or even the ones you settled into last year, or possibly last week.

It will be helpful to stay open to new interpretations of the world and how it might work. Often we get stuck in our current thinking because, like an old shoe, it is so comfortable. Move out of your comfort zone from time to time, and keep an open mind.

Stop Worrying

Worry, like negative thinking, is a habit. And, like negative thinking or any other habit, it can be broken once we become aware of it. But worry is sometimes so subtle and so insidious and so pervasive in our society, that we can worry for years and not even be aware of it.

I learned this lesson a few years back when I had completed a major project. After months of long, hard work and many sleepless nights (when I would lie awake worrying if everything would be all right,) finally the deadline was met and the project was completed. There was not a single thing more I could possibly do to make it better.

But one night a few weeks later, before I had a chance to start another project, I realized I was still waking in the middle of the night and lying there worrying about my completed project, even though there was nothing at all to worry about. Perhaps this same thing has happened to you.

As I lay there, I had one of those experiences we all have from time to time. I saw in a flash that I have been moving through life from one worry to the next. I examined each of the circumstances as I could remember them, and it became clear that not only had there never been anything to worry about, but worrying had never served any useful function. It was a total waste of energy that kept me from experiencing the joy of the moment and from getting any real sense of accomplishment from my work.

A worry-free life is incredibly liberating, and it will help you achieve inner peace.

Take Responsibility for Your life

There are those who say that, metaphysically, we choose all the circumstances of our life — our parents, our health, our physical characteristics, our race, and our cultural and geographical orientation, before we are born, and that we come into this life knowing, at some level, that we have to use those circumstances for our inner growth.

I do not know whether this is true, though I like to believe it is. But I do know that if I see my life as my responsibility, then I can make the changes necessary to create what I want and need to be happy.

If I take the position that someone else — a supreme power or whoever — is in charge and will take care of everything, I could be stuck for ages in circumstances I am not happy about and feel powerless to change them. I have learned that if there is something in my life that does not work, and I am waiting for someone else to fix it, I had better not be holding my breath.

Nowhere is this more applicable than in the inner realms. If you are already taking responsibility for the outer areas of your life, it will be easier to make the choices you need to make for your spiritual growth.

Accept the Things You Cannot Change

Taking responsibility for your life also means accepting the things you cannot change.

If you are short and want to be tall, or you are an endomorph and wish you were an ectomorph, if you were born with some impediment or acquired one along the way, or if you find yourself in any particular set of circumstances that are absolute, immutable, and irreversible, then you basically have two options. You can rant and rave and curse and indulge in remorse or guilt or self-pity. Or you can go along and deal with the situation and play the game the best you can.

You can be open to the possibility that those who say we have chosen our circumstances are correct, and then set about figuring out what you can learn from your life by making the most of it.

When you look at the personal limitations someone like Helen Keller had to deal with, and the extent to which she overcame them, not to mention the tremendous contribution she made with her life, you can see that it is possible to fight with the inescapable.

Going within to find the meaning of our life does not mean seeking to avoid the challenges our circumstances present. Rather it means finding the grace to learn how to live our lives to the fullest extent possible — whatever that is for us —

and, in the acceptance, to move on to the highest level of growth we can.

Get Comfortable with Change

Growth by definition requires change.

If you have spent years with certain habits, beliefs, and ways of doing things, inner growth may cause some upheaval in your life. Do not be put off by that. Get comfortable with it. Welcome it. Change offers an exciting, often exhilarating way of getting in touch with your soul.

But if you find yourself stuck in outdated habits and ways of operating that no longer serve you, spend some time thinking about how you might do things differently. True inner growth might well require that you experience new thoughts, new feelings, new sensations, new friendships, possibly even a new identity. Allow yourself to be vulnerable, and open yourself to change.

Get Out of Relationships that Do Not Support You

We humans, for the most part, still maintain our herd instincts. It is comforting to be one of the pack, and to have family, friends, and loved ones nearby to help us grow, at least at the start of our journey.

But it sometimes happens that the people we are closest to, do not really support us. Look around you, not just at your spouse and the family members you are involved with, but at all the relationships and associations you have in your life.

The lack of support can be so subtle. We can hang out for years with someone we love and think of as a friend before we begin to realize that the relationship is not really helping us and, in fact, has been holding us back.

It is easy to be deceived by the comfort a long-time relationship appears to offer you. There is a certain ease that comes with familiarity and from knowing each other's history, and from the history the two of you have built together, even when it has been tumultuous.

But there comes a time when you have to ask some hard questions: Does that person really love you, or are they hanging on to you because of their own lack or their own needs? They may say they love you, but do they make you feel loved? Are they really happy with you in your successes, or do they always manage to put you in the wrong? Do they love you enough to let you go on to bigger and better things, even if it means they get left behind?

Non-acceptance and subtle put-downs can be powerful deterrents to your growth. If you are not getting the love and support you need from the relationships in your life, it will be much harder for you to achieve inner happiness.

If you are moving on, sometimes there is really no choice but to leave behind those who may not be ready to move on with you.

Often you simply have to retreat with a smile, and gradually but resolutely reduce their presence in your life.

Realize that all the family ties and friendships in your life are there for a purpose, but they are not necessarily meant to last forever. It takes a certain grace to recognize when the time for a disabling relationship is over and, even if the other person does not recognize it, to bow out and move on. You will then have the time and energy to concentrate on loving, supportive relationships.

Explore Meditation

Meditation is one of the most powerful tools we have for self-expansion and inner growth. Through meditation we can reach levels of mental clarity that we cannot achieve through any other means. Meditation is a major pathway to the soul.

There are many ways to meditate. You can meditate on the inflow and outflow of the breath. You can meditate using a sacred word or phrase. You can meditate on the flame of a candle, or on the inner light at the centre of your forehead.

You can meditate on the idea of love, or wisdom, or immortality, or any other concept. Or you can meditate by simply being aware of your thoughts as they pass through your mind. There are sitting, standing, walking, laughing, crying, dancing, and chanting meditations. You can live every single moment of the day and night as meditation. And this is just for starters.

If you have not explored meditation, I urge you to consider it. Making meditation a regular part of your life will open you up to new and exciting possibilities for your inner growth.

If you do not know where to begin, start with one of the books on the subject and branch out from there. Or connect with a teacher, or contact people who have had experience with meditation. If you start now, you will be amazed, when you look back six months or a year from now, at how far you have come and by how much your life has changed for the better. You will also see how subtly you have been guided through the inner maze.

Meditation provides a natural unfolding of the process of inner exploration. Some of the rewards are immediate. Others take time, often years, to achieve. There is no substitute for simply doing it, and seeing what the rewards are for you.

Create Joy in Your Life

We all have special moments in our lives. They are available to us in one degree or another every single day. We can find them in the smile of someone we love, or in the smile of someone we do not even know. We can find them in the hug of a child, in the presence of a friend, or the touch of a lover.

Think about the times in your life when you have been overcome with joy. It is in those moments that you were in love with yourself and everyone else. It was in those moments you believed you could conquer the world.

It is from that imagination and that belief and that love that we can create our lives.

Think about the things that bring you joy, then make a point of connection with as many of them as possible and as often as possible. Tap into moments of joy again and again, and absorb it into your present moment.

TITLES IN THE SERIES

All You Wanted to Know About

Happiness

Relaxation

Spirituality

Self-Motivation

Spiritual Healing

Love & Relationships